Evaluation of Exposure to Tuberculosis Among Employees at a Long-term Care Facility

Marie A. de Perio, MD
R. Todd Niemeier, MS, CIH

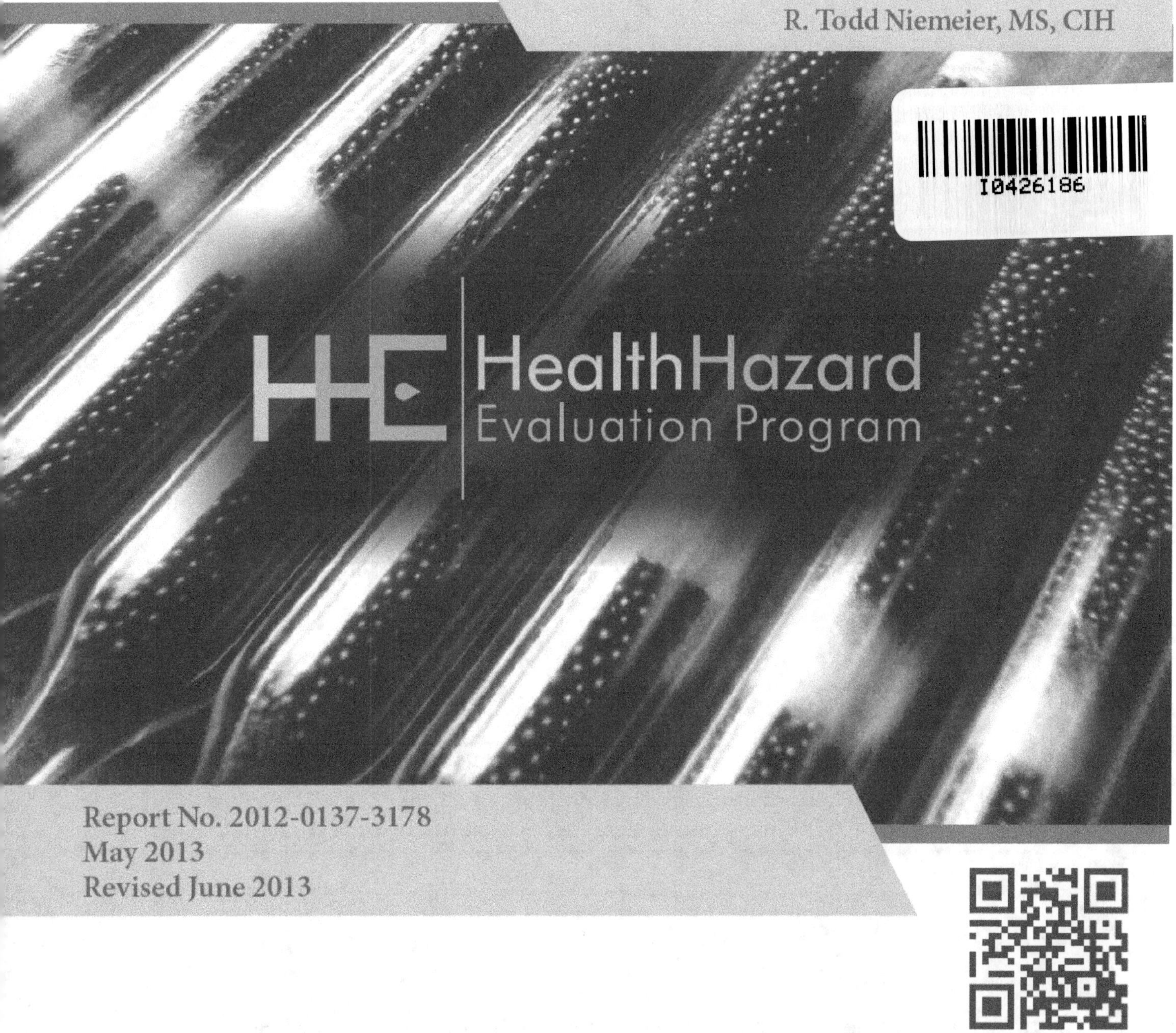

HealthHazard Evaluation Program

I0426186

Report No. 2012-0137-3178
May 2013
Revised June 2013

U.S. Department of Health and Human Services
Centers for Disease Control and Prevention
National Institute for Occupational Safety and Health

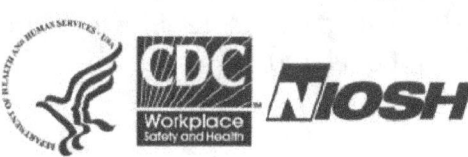

Contents

Revision Summary: The original final report contained inconsistent recommmentations about the frequency of tuberculin skin tests and medical evaluations for employees. The revised report notes that both should be done every 6 months until a risk assessment shows they can be done less often.

The employer is required to post a copy of this report for 30 days at or near the workplace(s) of affected employees. The employer must take steps to ensure that the posted report is not altered, defaced, or covered by other material.

The cover photo is a close-up image of sorbent tubes, which are used by the HHE Program to measure airborne exposures. This photo is an artistic representation that may not be related to this Health Hazard Evaluation.

Highlights of this Evaluation

The Health Hazard Evaluation Program received a request from a long-term care facility in Alaska. Managers were concerned about employee exposure to *Mycobacterium tuberculosis*. They asked for our assistance in identifying active tuberculosis disease sources and in assessing the ventilation system.

What We Did

- We visited the long-term care facility in May 2012 and August 2012.
- We interviewed 216 employees and reviewed employee health records.
- We reviewed pertinent medical records for 53 south side residents.
- We evaluated the ventilation system in some areas.

What We Found

- We found evidence of tuberculosis transmission among residents and employees.
- We found 12 residents and 16 employees who had latent tuberculosis infection.
- One resident with active pulmonary tuberculosis disease in the secure access unit was identified in late May 2012.
- This resident's active pulmonary tuberculosis disease is likely the source of the latent tuberculosis infection among the 8 secure access unit residents and the 16 employees.
- It is unclear whether this resident's active pulmonary tuberculosis disease is the source of the latent tuberculosis infection in the four south side residents.
- No clear pattern between the ventilation system and tuberculosis transmission was observed.

> We examined the recent incidence of active tuberculosis and latent tuberculosis infection among residents and employees at a long-term care facility. We also assessed the ventilation system. One resident with active pulmonary tuberculosis disease was identified, and healthcare-associated transmission of tuberculosis to 16 employees likely occurred in 2011–2012. Regular tuberculosis screening for residents and employees should continue.

What the Employer Can Do

- Provide annual tuberculosis training to all employees. Offer this training during work hours.
- Monitor south side residents clinically for signs and symptoms of active tuberculosis disease at least once a month.
- Continue tuberculosis screening of all south side residents, employees, and direct care volunteers at least every 6 months until a risk assessment shows it can be done less often.

What the Employer Can Do (continued)

- Upgrade the ventilation system to provide improved filters in resident areas according to current guidelines.

- Keep air temperatures according to current guidelines for nursing homes.

What Employees Can Do

- Get a tuberculin skin test at least every six months (or annually, according to the employer's schedule) if you had a negative tuberculin skin test in the past.

- Get a medical evaluation for tuberculosis at least every six months (or annually, according to the employer's schedule) if you had a positive tuberculin skin test in the past.

- Look for tuberculosis symptoms (cough $\geq$ 3 weeks duration, bloody sputum, night sweats, unexplained weight loss, unexplained fever) in residents and report these to the nursing supervisor and caring physician.

Mention of any company or product does not constitute endorsement by NIOSH. In addition, citations to websites external to NIOSH do not constitute NIOSH endorsement of the sponsoring organizations or their programs or products. Furthermore, NIOSH is not responsible for the content of these websites. All web addresses referenced in this document were accessible as of the publication date of this report.

Abbreviations

AFB	Acid fast bacilli
AHU	Air handling unit
AKDHSS	Alaska Department of Health and Social Services
ANSI	American National Standards Institute
ASHRAE	American Society of Heating, Refrigerating, and Air-Conditioning Engineers
CDC	Centers for Disease Control and Prevention
CFR	Code of Federal Regulations
CNA	Certified nursing assistant
CO_2	Carbon dioxide
IEQ	Indoor environmental quality
MERV	Minimum efficiency reporting value
PCR	Polymerase chain reaction
QFT-GIT	QuantiFERON®-TB Gold In-Tube test
RH	Relative humidity
TB	Tuberculosis
TST	Tuberculin skin test

Introduction

The Health Hazard Evaluation Program received a request from managers at a long-term care facility in Alaska. The request concerned the exposure of employees to *Mycobacterium tuberculosis*. The requestors asked for our assistance in identifying active tuberculosis (TB) disease sources and in assessing the ventilation system.

During on-site evaluations in May 2012 and August 2012, we observed workplace conditions and work processes and practices. We interviewed employees, reviewed employee health records and pertinent medical records for employees and residents, and evaluated the ventilation system in selected areas.

Tuberculosis

TB, a disease caused by the bacteria *Mycobacterium tuberculosis*, is spread from person to person through the air. TB usually infects the lungs but can also infect other body parts such as the brain, kidneys, or spine. The symptoms of active TB disease in any body part include feeling sick or weak, weight loss, fever, and night sweats. The symptoms of TB disease of the lungs also include coughing, chest pain, and coughing up blood.

TB bacteria are released into the air when a person with TB disease of the lungs or throat coughs, sneezes, speaks, or sings. These bacteria can stay in the air for several hours, depending on the environment. Persons who breathe air containing these TB bacteria can become infected.

Persons with latent TB infection have TB bacteria in their bodies, but they are not ill because the bacteria are not active. These persons do not have symptoms of TB disease, and they cannot spread the bacteria to others. They may develop TB disease in the future but can be treated to prevent this from happening. Persons with TB disease are sick from active TB bacteria when the bacteria are multiplying, which destroys tissues in their body. They usually have symptoms of TB disease and are capable of spreading TB bacteria to others.

Long-term Care Facility

At the time of our visits, the long-term care facility was an approximately 48,000-square foot, 190-bed center providing skilled care and rehabilitation services to its residents. It was part of a large network of healthcare facilities operated by a local organization. The original building was constructed in the 1960s. Since then, additional wings and community rooms had been added to the building. The center was physically separated into four "neighborhoods" on the basis of individual resident needs. The "south side" of the building had two neighborhoods (Chugach and Denali neighborhoods) and a restricted access area specializing in the care of residents with dementia and other cognitive dysfunction (secure access unit). As of August 2010, the secure access unit had a 24 licensed bed capacity. As of August 2011, the secure access unit had a 15 licensed bed capacity. Residents of the secure access unit had limited interaction with residents in other neighborhoods. The "north side" of the building had two additional neighborhoods, Mat-su and the transitional care unit. Starting in January 2013, residents on the south side of the building began to be moved to a newly constructed facility. Eventually, only the transitional care unit will remain in the current facility.

Each neighborhood had a large dining room where residents were encouraged to eat their meals, and each resident room accommodated two people. The facility had approximately 330 employees and 140 residents at the time of our visits. In May 2012, 66 residents lived on the south side, including 11 residents in the secure access unit. In August 2012, 65 residents lived on the south side, including the same 11 residents in the secure access unit.

Visitors and volunteers regularly spent time with residents in the facility. Length of stay for residents varied from a few weeks to many years. The facility had no airborne infection isolation rooms. Residents requiring airborne infection isolation were transferred to the facility's affiliated hospital or other area acute care facilities within 5 hours of recognition.

According to the facility's tuberculosis plan as of February 2012, individuals seeking admission to the facility had to be free of signs and symptoms of active TB disease. All residents without a history of TB or a positive tuberculin skin test (TST) were screened for TB within 72 hours of admission followed by a second step TST 7–10 days later. Residents then received a TST annually during the month of their admission anniversary. Residents with a history of active TB disease or positive TST were screened for TB by questionnaire.

Also according to the facility's tuberculosis plan, employees received TB screening prior to their first day at work through the employee health office. Employees then completed annual TB screening during the month of their birthday. Prior to this and related investigations, employees were screened annually every April. The facility had not experienced any TST conversions among employees or residents during annual TB screening the previous several years.

Prior Related Investigations

During the facility's annual TB screening in April 2011, eight employees were found to have a TST conversion (a new positive TST result after having previously negative TST results). All eight employees provided direct care to the residents of the secure access unit; most also provided care to residents of other neighborhoods. Around that time, four of the 17 residents of the secure access unit were found to have positive QuantiFERON®-TB Gold In-Tube test (QFT-GIT) results after having previously negative TST results. An investigation by the facility, the Alaska Department of Health and Social Services (AKDHSS), and the municipal health department identified no current residents or employees (as of April 2011) with active TB disease.

Follow-up TB screening in July 2011–October 2011 found four additional residents in the secure access unit with new positive QFT-GIT results after having a previous negative QFT-GIT result. In addition, during this time, seven additional employees were found to have new positive QFT-GIT results after having a previous negative QFT-GIT result.

In November 2011, AKDHSS, with assistance from the Division of TB Elimination at the Centers for Disease Control and Prevention (CDC), investigated the epidemiology of TB at the facility and attempted to identify active TB sources. Investigators screened 143 employees who spent at least some time in the secure access unit using a combination of interviews, a chest radiograph, and TST. They also reviewed medical records for 32 current and former unit residents during the exposure period of concern, January 2010–November 2011. At the conclusion of that field visit, no employees or residents had been identified as an active TB disease source. Investigators recommended continuing to identify and treat active TB disease and latent TB infection, including specific recommendations for clinical evaluation of unit residents.

In March–April 2012, repeat TB screening identified one employee and four residents with new positive TST results. The employee, a certified nursing assistant, had a primary assignment in the south side of the building, and the four residents lived in the south side of the building outside of the secure access unit.

To supplement the facility's ongoing investigation, managers at the facility asked the Health Hazard Evaluation Program for assistance in identifying active TB disease sources and in assessing the ventilation system.

Assessment

The purpose of our evaluation was to (1) investigate the incidence of active TB disease and latent TB infection among facility employees and residents; (2) assess the facility's ventilation system; and (3) recommend ways to improve TB-related occupational health and infection control practices.

We observed workplace conditions and work processes and practices and spoke with employees. We focused our epidemiologic investigation on the south side of the building because that was where the employee and four residents with recent TST conversions were located. We held confidential medical interviews with employees, reviewed pertinent employee health records, and reviewed resident medical records. We also cross-checked names of residents, volunteers, and visitors with the Alaska state TB disease database. Also, we evaluated the ventilation systems in the building.

Confidential Medical Interviews and Medical Record Review of Employees

At our request, facility staff grouped current and former employees (those whose employment terminated January 2012–August 2012) into three risk categories: (1) employees with a primary assignment in the south side of the building, (2) employees who spent some time on the south side of the building, and (3) employees who were not known to spend any time on the south side of the building.

Facility staff identified 61 category 1 employees (57 current and 4 former employees), 179 category 2 employees (163 current and 16 former employees), and 110 category 3 employees (103 current and 7 former employees). We selected all 240 category 1 and 2 employees to participate in individual, semistructured confidential interviews during our two visits or by telephone. During these interviews completed May 21, 2012–August 23, 2012, we discussed employees' pertinent medical history, their work history including time spent on the south side of the building, and any current active TB disease symptoms. We asked if they recalled having been in contact with any residents, coworkers, or visitors with signs of TB disease.

We supplemented the information gathered from these interviews with information from employee health and other pertinent medical records. This information included TB screening information such as history of TB disease or latent TB infection, results of TST or QFT-GIT testing, chest radiographs, and acid fast bacilli (AFB) sputum samples.

Resident Medical Record Review

During both visits, we also reviewed electronic medical records for 53 south side residents in the Chugach and Denali neighborhoods and one deceased resident from the south side. This total excluded the 11 secure access unit residents and one recently arrived resident. We abstracted information on demographic, social, and medical characteristics, including TB risk factors and signs and symptoms suggestive of active TB disease. We also arranged a clinical consultative conference on May 23, 2012, with colleagues from the CDC Division of TB Elimination who provided direct recommendations to the medical director regarding the further clinical evaluation of some residents.

Crosscheck with Alaska State Tuberculosis Database

During our first visit, a nurse epidemiologist from the Division of Public Health in AKDHSS compared the list of 53 residents present in the south side as of May 13, 2012, with the state TB disease database dating back to the early 1970s. We also obtained a list of volunteers with direct resident contact and the visitor log sheets from November 2011 to the date of our visit. The nurse epidemiologist from AKDHSS also compared these lists of names with the state TB disease database.

Ventilation Assessment

We walked through the resident areas, mechanical rooms, and roof top to observe the ventilation system. We also reviewed ventilation plans with the engineering staff. We obtained airflow measurements from supply diffusers and ducted returns in 14 resident rooms and adjoining bathrooms in each of the four neighborhoods on the north and south sides of the building using a TSI VelociCalc Plus® thermoanemometer (TSI, Inc., Shoreview, Minnesota). We used smoke tubes to visualize airflow in the doorways for these resident rooms relative to adjacent hallways.

Additional Indoor Environmental Quality Assessment

General indoor environmental quality (IEQ) data (carbon dioxide [CO_2] concentrations and temperature and relative humidity [RH] levels) were collected over a 24-hour period at four nursing stations in the four neighborhoods using TSI Q-Trak™ Plus instruments (TSI, Inc., Shoreview, Minnesota) to evaluate general ventilation and occupant comfort indicators. These comfort indicators provide information about the functioning and control of HVAC systems. We also collected spot measurements for temperature, RH, and CO_2 in the minimum dataset office located in the transitional care unit because of an employee complaint that the area was "stuffy." Finally, the facility provided information on the history of the rooms that residents with TST conversions on the south side and secure access unit were housed in since 2010 as well as a list of the roommates of these residents.

Results

Confidential Medical Interviews and Medical Record Review of Employees

Using lists generated by facility staff, we interviewed 58 (95%) of the 61 current or former category 1 employees and 158 (88%) of the 179 current or former category 2 employees. The 24 category 1 and 2 employees (16 current and 8 former) who were not interviewed were not working during our visits, were unreachable by telephone, or did not have current contact information.

The 216 interviewed employees included 118 (83%) of the 143 employees screened during the investigation by CDC and AKDHSS in November 2011 and 98 employees not screened during that investigation.

After reviewing self-reported locations worked by those employees interviewed, we reclassified some employees into different risk categories on the basis of their reported work locations. Therefore, of the 216 employees, we interviewed 86 current or former category 1 employees, 114 current or former category 2 employees, and 16 category 3 employees.

Work Characteristics

Of the 216 interviewed employees, the median number of years worked at the facility was 5 years (range: 6 weeks–32 years). The median number of hours worked per week was 40 hours (range: 8–60 hours). Other work characteristics of interviewed employees are shown in Table 1.

Table 1. Work characteristics of interviewed employees

Work characteristic	No. (%) interviewed employees n = 216
Job title*	
Certified nursing assistant	81 (38)
Supervisory nurse, registered nurse, or licensed practical nurse	59 (27)
Environmental services	19 (9)
Physical, occupational, or speech therapist	12 (6)
Dietary/nutrition services	8 (4)
Laundry services	6 (3)
Activities therapist	5 (2)
Respiratory therapist	5 (2)
Physician or nurse practitioner	3 (1)
Other	18 (8)
Self-reported resident contact	
Direct resident care/close contact	177 (82)
Brief encounters	30 (14)
No contact with residents	9 (4)
Work shift†	
Day	128 (59)
Evening	52 (24)
Night	30 (14)
Various	6 (3)

*Job title of current employees at the time of interview or job title of former employees during employment at the facility

†Work shift of current employees at the time of interview or work shift of former employees during employment at the facility

Tuberculosis Risk Factors

During the interviews, we asked employees if they had any TB risk factors. Of the 216 interviewed employees, 166 (77%) reported at least one TB risk factor. Of the 216 interviewed employees, 110 (51%) were foreign born, and 100 (46%) reported having received the Bacillus Calmette-Guérin (BCG) vaccine. Other TB risk factors are shown in Table 2. Diabetes mellitus was the most common TB risk factor (12% of interviewed employees).

Table 2. Tuberculosis risk factors of interviewed employees

Characteristic	No. (%) interviewed employees n = 216
Foreign-born	110 (51)
Philippines	74 (34)
Palau	5 (2)
Laos	5 (2)
Dominica	4 (2)
American Samoa	4 (2)
Other	18 (8)
Residence or work in another long-term care facility	66 (31)
Residence or work in correctional facility	5 (2)
Homelessness	3 (1)
Diabetes mellitus	26 (12)
Other*	4 (2)

*Other includes taking immunosuppressive medication, severe kidney disease, and illicit drug use.

Tuberculosis Screening Record

We reviewed TB screening records of all 240 category 1 and 2 employees identified by the facility. Of the 216 interviewed employees, only one reported a history of ever being treated for TB disease. This foreign born registered nurse reported being treated for presumptive TB disease with four-drug therapy in 1986 during nursing school in a country with high prevalence of TB after her father was diagnosed with TB disease. She had a chest radiograph that reportedly showed no signs of TB disease in November 2011. The nurse also had two sputum samples collected in May 2012, both of which were AFB smear negative and AFB culture negative. During the interview in August 2012, the nurse denied any symptoms of TB disease since January 2011.

Other TB screening results of interviewed and noninterviewed employees are shown in Table 3. Of the 216 interviewed employees, 60 (28%) had a history of a positive TST either by report or on hire. Nine (4%) employees had TST conversions in 2011, all of whom were thought to be part of the cluster at the center of the prior investigations. Of these, six employees were found to have positive QFT-GIT results, one was found to have a negative QFT-GIT, and two did not have QFT-GIT testing. Forty-four employees reported current or previous treatment for latent TB infection (Table 3).

Table 3. Tuberculosis screening of employees

Screening	No. (%) employees interviewed n = 216	No. (%) employees not interviewed n = 24
TST positive		
Before 2011*	60 (28)	4 (17)
Conversion in 2011	9 (4)†	0 (0)
Conversion in 2012	1 (0.5)‡	0 (0)
QFT-GIT positive	45 (21)§	1 (4)¶
Current or previous treatment for latent TB infection	44 (20)	1 (4)
Chest radiograph performed**		
Since November 1, 2011	111 (51)	9 (38)
Since April 1, 2011	133 (62)	5 (21)
Submitted adequate sputum sample May 2012††		
At least 1 sample	162 (75)	7 (29)
At least 2 samples	124 (57)	4 (17)
Did not have chest radiograph since April 1, 2011 or sputum sample May 2012	17 (8)‡‡	12 (50)§§

*TST positivity by report or found on hire

†Six of these employees were found to have positive QFT-GIT results, 1 was found to have negative QFT-GIT results, and 2 did not have QFT-GIT testing results.

‡This employee was found to have a positive QFT-GIT result.

§All of these employees also had a positive TST result, and this included the employee with a TST conversion in 2012 and 6 employees with TST conversions in 2011.

¶This employee reported a positive TST prior to employment.

**All chest radiographs were reported to be negative for signs of TB disease.

††All sputum samples collected from employees were reported to be AFB smear negative and AFB culture negative.

‡‡Fifteen of these 17 employees were current employees.

§§Eight of these 12 employees were current employees.

One employee was found to have a TST conversion in 2012. This employee was a U.S. born certified nursing assistant (CNA) who worked primarily in the south side of the building and also spent time in the secure access unit. The employee had a negative two-step TST on hire in January 2012 and was found to have a TST conversion in March 2012. The employee denied a history of active TB disease symptoms and had no known risk factors for progression to active TB disease. The employee's chest radiograph showed no signs of active TB disease. This employee began treatment for latent TB infection in April 2012.

Employees underwent various TB screening modalities in 2011–2012. Of the 203 current employees interviewed, all 135 with no prior history of a positive TST or QFT-GIT underwent either TST or QFT-GIT screening in 2012. Also, 133 (62%) of the interviewed employees had a chest radiograph since April 2011 as part of the previous investigations at the facility. In addition, prior to our first site visit, the facility, in conjunction with the AKDHSS, collected sputum samples from current employees during the first week of May 2012. Employees unable to give sputum during that week were encouraged to have sputum samples collected at the municipal health department. In total, 162 (75%) of interviewed employees submitted at least one sputum sample. In total, 257 of all current category 1, 2, and 3 employees submitted at least one adequate sputum sample in May 2012. All sputum samples collected from employees were reported to be AFB smear negative and AFB culture negative.

Of the 24 category 1 and 2 employees unable to be interviewed, four (17%) had a history of a positive TST either by report or on hire (Table 3). Only one was known to have been treated for latent TB infection. All four had chest radiographs performed since April 2011. Two had at least one sputum sample collected, and all samples were reported to be negative on AFB smear and negative on AFB culture.

In June 2012–August 2012, TB screening of 214 employees revealed no new TST conversions. In September 2012–October 2012, TB screening of 191 employees revealed no new TST conversions.

Tuberculosis Signs and Symptoms

We asked employees if they had any TB disease signs and symptoms (including productive cough for $\geq$ 3 weeks, unexpected weight loss, persistent fever > 100°F, night sweats, loss of appetite, coughing up blood, fatigue or weakness, or hoarseness) since January 2011. Seven employees reported at least two of these symptoms. Four of the seven attributed them to diagnoses including diabetes mellitus, adrenal sufficiency, menopause, and sinusitis.

Of the three employees reporting symptoms that could be consistent with TB and with no other known alternate diagnoses, all were U.S. born. One CNA, who was no longer working at the facility upon interview in July 2012, reported a history of chronic symptoms, including cough and night sweats, over the previous 3 months. She reported seeing her personal physician during this time and being diagnosed with bronchitis. The CNA had a previously negative TST in July 2011, and a normal chest radiograph in November 2011. She was no longer an employee of the center when sputum collection occurred in May 2012. After the telephone interview, we recommended further clinical evaluation at the municipal health department.

Another CNA, who was still working at the center upon interview in May 2012, reported symptoms including fever, cough, weight loss, and loss of appetite, which had intermittently recurred over the previous 3 months. She reported seeing her personal physician during this time and being diagnosed with influenza. This CNA had a previously negative TST in February 2012, and had one sputum sample, collected in May 2012, which had a negative AFB smear and negative AFB culture. We also recommended she obtain further clinical evaluation.

Another employee, working in environmental services, upon interview in August 2012, reported symptoms including cough, weakness, and hoarseness over the previous 3 weeks.

He reported seeing his personal physician and being diagnosed with bronchitis. This employee had a previously negative TST in June 2012, a normal chest radiograph in November 2011, and two sputum samples collected in May 2012, which had negative AFB smears and negative AFB cultures. We also recommended he obtain further clinical evaluation.

Resident Medical Record Review

During both visits, we reviewed electronic medical records for 53 south side residents and one deceased resident who had been located in the south side. The median age of the residents was 62 years (range: 23–94 years); 28 (52%) were male. Identified races included White (n = 33, 61%), Alaska Native (n = 9, 17%), Black/African American (n = 7, 13%), Asian (n = 4, 7%), and unknown (n = 1, 2%).

Tuberculosis Risk Factors

We reviewed each south side resident's TB risk factors. Diabetes mellitus was the most common TB risk factor (44% of residents). Other TB risk factors are shown in Table 4. Country of birth was not documented for 37 (70%) of the residents in their medical records.

Table 4. Tuberculosis risk factors of facility residents

Characteristic	No. (%) residents n = 54
Foreign-born	5 (9)
Germany	2 (4)
Philippines	1 (2)
South Korea	1 (2)
Vietnam	1 (2)
Diabetes mellitus	24 (44)
HIV infection or taking immunosuppressive medication	1 (2)
Severe kidney disease	3 (6)
Illicit drug or excess alcohol use	5 (9)

Tuberculosis Screening Records

We reviewed TB screening records of 54 south side residents. Only one of the 54 residents had a history of TB disease, and this occurred prior to admission to the facility. At the time of the evaluation, this resident was reported to have a chronic productive cough without any other TB symptoms. The resident had a chest radiograph in July 2012, which showed no signs of TB disease. The resident also had one sputum sample collected in May 2012, which was AFB smear negative and AFB culture negative.

Other TB screening results of the 54 south side residents are shown in Table 5. Of these, 7 (13%) had a history of a positive TST either by report or on admission. Only one of these 7 residents was reported to have undergone latent TB infection treatment.

Table 5. Tuberculosis screening of south side residents

Screening	No. (%) south side residents n = 54
TST positive	
Before 2012*	7 (13)
Conversion in 2012	4 (7)†
Current or previous treatment for latent TB infection	4 (7)
Chest radiograph performed‡	
Since November 1, 2011	28 (52)
Since April 1, 2011	37 (69)
Submitted adequate sputum sample since May 2012§	
At least 1 sample¶	17 (31)
At least 2 samples¶	10 (19)
Submitted stool sample for TB polymerase chain reaction (PCR)	5 (9)
Did not have chest radiograph since April 1, 2011, or sputum sample since May 2012**	12 (22)

*TST positivity by report or found on admission

†Three of these residents were found to have positive QFT-GIT results; 1 was found to have negative QFT-GIT result.

‡All chest radiographs were reported to negative for signs of TB disease.

§All sputum samples collected from residents were reported to be AFB smear negative and AFB culture negative.

¶Nine residents had tracheal aspirates sent for AFB testing.

**All stool samples had reportedly negative TB PCR results.

Four (7%) of the 54 south side residents had a documented TST conversion in 2012. Of these, three residents were also found to have positive QFT-GIT results, and one was found to have a negative QFT-GIT result. The TB risk factors for resident 1, in addition to residing in a long-term care facility, included Type II diabetes mellitus, which was fairly well controlled. The resident's TB symptoms included a 1-year history of weight loss. The computed tomography scans for resident 1 from March 2012 and July 2012 showed no evidence of TB disease in the lungs. Three sputum samples were collected in July 2012, which were all AFB smear negative and AFB culture negative. Shortly after this sputum was collected, resident 1 was started on isoniazid therapy for latent TB infection treatment.

The additional TB risk factors of the second resident with a TST conversion, resident 2, included end-stage renal disease requiring hemodialysis. Resident 2 had no reported TB symptoms. A chest radiograph obtained in April 2012 showed stable left lung granulomas but no evidence of TB disease. Sputum was unable to be collected from the resident; rifampin was started in August 2012.

The third resident with a TST conversion, resident 3, did not have any apparent additional TB risk factors and also had no reported TB symptoms. A chest radiograph obtained in April 2012 showed no evidence of TB disease. The resident was unable to produce sputum for analysis and had not been started on latent TB infection therapy as of our second visit in August 2012.

The fourth resident with a TST conversion, resident 4, had no known additional TB risk factors beyond being an Alaska native. A QFT-GIT obtained in May 2012 was negative. The reported TB symptoms of resident 4 included weight loss, loss of appetite, and a productive cough. A chest radiograph obtained in April 2012 showed evidence of right-sided pulmonary nodules, some of which were calcified, but no evidence of TB disease. A computed tomography of the chest in May 2012 showed no evidence of lung disease. Resident 4 was unable to produce sputum. A stool TB PCR test and urine AFB smears and cultures were all negative in May 2012. The resident was started on rifampin shortly thereafter but died in August 2012 due to respiratory failure. No postmortem examination was done.

All of the 42 south side residents, who had no prior history of TB disease or a positive TST or QFT-GIT, underwent TST screening on multiple dates in 2012. Also, 28 (52%) of the 54 south side residents had a chest radiograph since November 2011. All were reported to be negative for signs of active TB disease. In addition, the facility collected at least one sputum or tracheal aspirate sample from 17 (31%) residents. All samples were reported to be AFB smear negative and AFB culture positive. The rest of the residents were unable to produce sputum for collection.

In July 2012 and again in October 2012, TB screening revealed no new TST or QFT-GIT conversions among south side residents.

Crosscheck with Alaska Tuberculosis Database

None of the 53 residents present in the south side as of May 13, 2012, matched with the Alaska TB disease database dating back to the early 1970s. None of the volunteers with direct resident contact nor the visitors who had signed the visitor log sheets from November 2011 to May 2012 matched with the state TB disease database.

Identification of Active Tuberculosis Disease in Resident

During our evaluation, we learned that a female resident in her 90s in the secure access unit was diagnosed with active TB disease. This resident had a history of advanced dementia and a remote history of active pulmonary TB disease. Her symptoms included a chronic productive cough since February 2011 and weight loss. The resident had an extensive work up dating back to April 2011. Her work up included a chest radiograph in April 2011 that showed scattered interstitial opacities. The resident then underwent a bronchoscopy in May 2011, and bronchoalveolar lavage fluid was reported to be AFB smear negative and AFB culture negative. A repeat chest radiograph in October 2011 was unchanged, and the resident's stool PCR for TB was negative in November 2011.

As part of the joint sputum collection effort by the facility and the AKDHSS, sputum was collected from this resident on May 7, 2012. The AFB smear was found to be negative, but the AFB culture was found to be positive on May 28, 2012. The isolate was identified to be *Mycobacterium tuberculosis*, genotype G15524, a genotype only found in Alaska. That same day, as per the facility's tuberculosis plan, dated February 2012, the resident was transferred to an acute care hospital. Another sputum sample collected on June 1, 2012, was reported to be AFB smear negative but AFB culture positive. This resident (the index resident) started four-drug treatment on June 1, 2012, and was transferred back to the facility on June 15, 2012.

Ventilation Assessment

At the time of our evaluation, the ventilation system was a constant air volume system, meaning that the supply air airflow rate remained steady throughout the day, but the

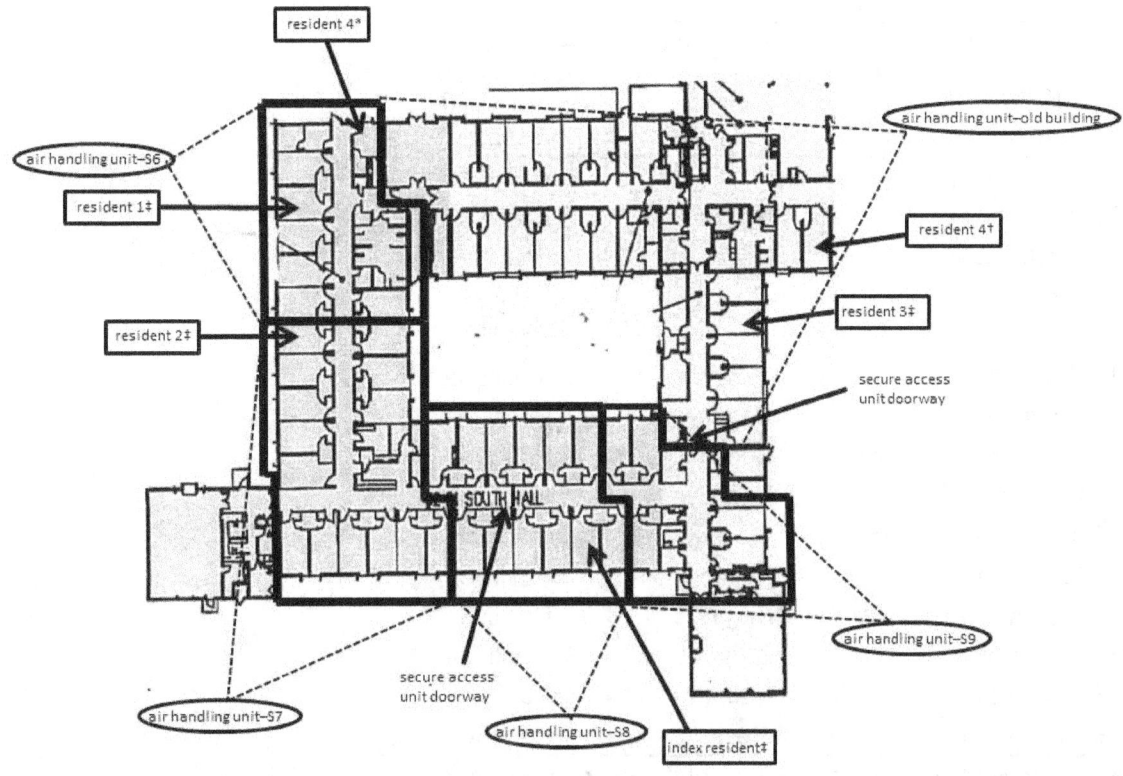

Figure 1. Map of south side of the long-term care facility.
*Resident 4 lived in this room from January 27, 2012–February 15, 2012.
†Resident 4 lived in this room from prior to February 2011 to January 23, 2012, and from February 15, 2012, until the dates of our site visit (May 2012).
‡Residents 1, 2, and 3 lived in these rooms from prior to February 2011 to the dates of our first site visit (May 2012).

temperature of the supply air varied to meet the thermal set points. Several air handling units (AHUs) served different parts of the building. Figure 1 shows a map of the south side of the building and the areas served by each AHU. Most of these perimeter units mixed air from the ducted returns with 40% outdoor air before supplying it back to the occupied areas. Outdoor air was passed through a set of minimum efficiency reporting value (MERV) 8 filters and mixed with return air before distribution. The oldest section of the building (center section on both the north and south sides) had a ventilation system that consisted of two AHUs that were single pass, meaning that all of the return air was exhausted from the building (no recirculation). A visual inspection of some of the AHUs serving the south side of the building revealed that these units appeared clean and well-maintained. No test and balance of the ventilation system had been completed since 1988.

Smoke tube testing found that some resident rooms were under negative pressure relative to the adjacent hallway (i.e., air was flowing from the adjacent hallway into the resident room), while other resident rooms were under positive pressure relative to the adjacent hallway (i.e., air was flowing from the resident room into the adjacent hallway). One resident room

Table 6. Direction of airflow between resident rooms and adjacent hallways and bathrooms on May 22, 2012, and May 23, 2012

Resident room	Air pressure relationship to adjacent hallway	Air pressure relationship to adjacent bathroom
125 (North side)	Negative	Bidirectional*
141 (North side)	Negative	Positive
167 (North side)	Negative	Positive
181 (North side)	Positive	Positive
207 (South side)	Positive	Positive
217 (South side)	Positive	Bidirectional*
223 (South Side)	Negative	Positive
228 (Secure access unit)	Negative	Positive
231 (Secure access unit)	Negative	Positive
235 (Secure access unit)	Positive	Not collected
257 (South side)	Negative	Positive
263 (South side)	Negative	Positive
267 (South side)	Neutral	Bidirectional*
273 (South side)	Negative	Positive
288 (South side)	Positive	Positive

*Airflow moved in different directions at the top and bottom of the doorway.

had neutral airflow to the adjacent hallway. These results are found in Table 6. ASHRAE does not provide recommendations for the pressure relationship between resident rooms and adjacent areas in skilled nursing facilities [ASHRAE 2011]. Most of the bathrooms within the resident rooms were under negative pressure relative to the resident room as expected due to the presence of exhaust fans in the bathrooms. However, we noted that for three of the resident rooms, airflow was in different directions along the doorway separating the resident room and bathroom. The bathroom exhaust fans were running in all of the bathrooms that we tested. In the two doorways separating the secure access unit from adjacent units, the smoke test revealed that air was moving from the adjacent units into the secure access unit on the day of our evaluation.

The secure access unit was in a newer section on the south side of the building and was served by two AHUs (AHU-S8 and AHU-S9). AHU-S8 also served part of the adjacent Denali unit. As described above, both of the AHUs serving the secure access unit recirculated air throughout the areas served by the ventilation system.

We had originally intended to collect airflow measurements at supply diffusers and ducted returns using an air capture hood in select resident rooms. However, this piece of equipment malfunctioned, and we instead used a thermoanemometer to collect these measurements. We are not reporting these measurements because turbulent airflow during the collection may have affected their accuracy.

We reviewed the index resident's room history compared to the other four residents with TB conversions to determine the likelihood of shared air space. The index resident lived in the same room in the secure access unit almost continuously from February 2011 through the dates of our site visit. This resident with active TB disease reportedly did not leave the secure access unit while residing there. She did have a brief stay in the north side of the building from June 23, 2011–July 13, 2011, before moving back to her room in the secure access unit. At the time of our site visit, three of the four residents with TST conversions (residents 1, 2, and 4) were located in adjacent hallways separated by locked doors to the index resident, with the closest resident (resident 2) located seven resident rooms away. Figure 1 shows the location of the four residents with TST conversions and the index resident when we made our site visit. Residents 1, 2, and 3 resided in these rooms from February 2011 through the dates of our site visit. Resident 4 lived in two rooms at separate times on the south side of the building. Resident 4 was located in one of these rooms from before February 2011–January 23, 2012, and in this same room from February 15, 2012, until the time of our site visit. This resident was also located in another room on the south side of the building from January 27, 2012–February 15, 2012. From the time period from January 23, 2012–January 27, 2012, resident 4 was located on the north side of the building.

During one period between April 2010 and May 2010, resident 2 was located diagonally across the hallway from the index resident, and their rooms shared the same ventilation system. However, because the index resident had cough and weight loss symptoms reported to start in February 2011, she was not likely infectious during this overlapping period. Resident 3 also had a negative TST documented in September 2011.

Additional Indoor Environmental Quality Assessment

The results of the IEQ data collection (temperature, RH, and CO_2) are provided in Table 7.

The CO_2 concentrations in four nursing stations were within guidelines recommended by the American National Standards Institute (ANSI)/ASHRAE [ANSI/ASHRAE 2011]. Spot CO_2

Table 7. Summary of IEQ data collected at nursing stations and minimum dataset office May 21 through May 22, 2012

Location	CO_2 concentration (parts per million)	Temp (°F)	RH (%)
Nursing station, Secure access unit	344–1029	74–83	23–34
Nursing station, Chugach	359–528	78–84	18–30
Nursing station, Transitional care unit	477–802	75–78	24–32
Nursing station, Mat-su	425–926	80–83	22–32
Minimum dataset office*	676	77	34
Outdoor	361–364	—	—

*Spot data collected at approximately 2:00 p.m. on May 22, 2012.

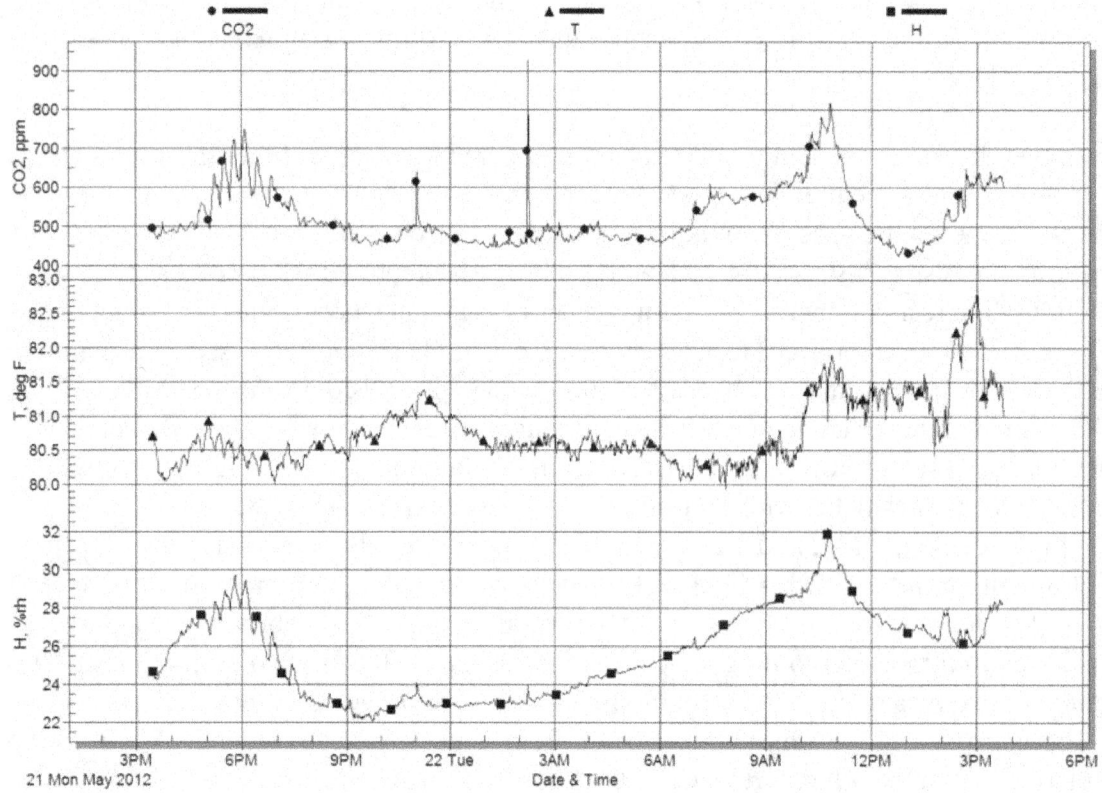

Figure 2. CO_2, temperature, and RH levels in the Mat-su unit collected May 21–22, 2012.

measurements collected in the minimum dataset office were also within ANSI/ASHRAE guidelines. Temperatures up to 84°F were measured, which generally exceeded the levels recommended by ASHRAE for nonresident areas in nursing facilities at the nursing stations and minimum dataset office [ASHRAE 2011]. All RH measurements were below 34%. ANSI/ASHRAE recommends that RH be maintained at or below 65% to minimize excessive growth of microorganisms and dust mites [ANSI/ASHRAE 2010a]. Figure 2 shows an example of the measurements collected in the Mat-su unit over a 24-hour period.

The minimum dataset office had three employees and was approximately 16 feet by 9.5 feet. Comfort parameter results are presented in Table 7. CO_2 levels were within ANSI/ASHRAE guidelines [ANSI/ASHRAE 2010b]. The temperature slightly exceeded ASHRAE guidelines for nonresident areas in nursing facilities [ASHRAE 2011]. The RH was 34%. The office had a supply diffuser and ducted return that appeared to be working when tested with a smoke tube, but there were no recent measurements of airflow rates. The office was under strong negative pressure relative to the adjacent hallway, indicating that more air was exhausted than supplied. The office employees reported that the "stuffiness" went away if the door to the hallway was left open. Reportedly, this door was usually left closed because of distracting noise from adjacent areas.

Discussion

Our evaluation, supported by prior investigations, revealed evidence of transmission of TB within the long-term care facility among residents and employees. In total, 12 residents and 16 employees were found to have latent TB infection by TST and/or QFT-GIT conversion. One resident with active pulmonary TB disease, likely secondary to reactivation, who resided in the secure access unit was identified in late May 2012. TB transmission from this resident likely explains the TST and QFT-GIT conversions among the eight secure access unit residents and the 16 employees. However, it is unclear whether this resident's active pulmonary TB disease was the source of exposure for the TST conversions seen in the four south side residents.

The secure access unit was served by two AHUs that mixed return air with 40% outdoor air. One of these units also served part of the adjacent Denali neighborhood. None of the four south side residents with TST conversions lived in rooms on the same ventilation systems as the resident with active TB disease in the secure access unit. However, because the ventilation system was not designed to control airborne infectious aerosols, it is possible that TB infectious aerosols could have migrated to other resident care areas. In addition, all but one of the three south side residents with TST conversions reportedly left their rooms and spent time in the hallways or in their common Denali or Chugach dining areas. Though it was observed that air moved into the secure access unit from both doorways leading to adjacent units on the day of our evaluation, many factors could influence the potential for shared air including opening and closing of resident room doors, opening or closing doors leading from the secure access unit to adjacent units, or opening exterior windows on either side of the doorways leading into the secure unit.

Subsequent TB screening by the facility in July 2012 and October 2012 revealed no additional TST or QFT-GIT conversions among employees and south side residents. This suggests that transmission appears to have stopped within the facility.

No active TB source was identified to definitively explain the TST conversions of the four south side residents. We identified, however, several possible explanations.

First, it is possible that one of the four residents with a TST conversion was actually a source of active TB disease. Three of these four residents were unable to have sputum collected for AFB analysis. Two of these three residents had no reported TB symptoms, and chest radiographs in April 2012 showed no evidence of active TB disease. However, the remaining resident did have a history of a productive cough, appetite loss, and weight loss. While a chest radiograph and computed tomography of the chest showed no evidence of active pulmonary TB disease, the resident died in August 2012, and no postmortem examination was done.

Second, it is also possible that one of the other south side residents was a source of active TB disease. While many of these residents underwent some clinical evaluation for TB, 12 (22%) of the 54 residents had neither a chest radiograph since April 1, 2011, nor a sputum sample since May 2012. Of these 12 residents, one resident, who was reported to have a productive cough and loss of appetite, died in April 2012.

Third, it is possible that an employee was the source of active TB disease. Extensive screening of employees by the facility and the AKDHSS, through interviews, TST, QFT-GIT, chest radiographs, and sputum collection for AFB analysis, revealed no active TB disease among any employees. Three (1%) of the 216 interviewed employees, however, reported symptoms consistent with TB. All were recommended to undergo further clinical evaluation. One of the three employees stopped working at the facility in May 2012, and this might explain the cessation in transmission.

Finally, it is also possible that a facility volunteer or visitor was the source of active TB disease. While a crosscheck of direct care volunteers and visitor names revealed no matches with the state TB disease database, it is possible that the potential source had not been diagnosed at that time or had been diagnosed in a different state. Visitor names in the log sheet were frequently illegible, making it difficult to crosscheck with the database. In addition, we were unable to obtain lists of volunteers not involved in direct care to crosscheck with the database.

In 2011, Alaska had the highest TB case rate of the 50 U.S. states at 9.3 cases per 100,000 persons [CDC 2012b]. In the United States, the incidence of TB has been higher in adults aged 65 years and older compared to the general population. In 2011, the TB case rate in adults aged 65 years and older was 5.4 cases per 100,000 persons compared to the national case rate of 3.4 cases per 100,000 persons [CDC 2012b]. Nursing home residence had been reported to double the age-adjusted risk of developing active TB disease [CDC 1990; Yoshikawa 1992]. The elderly population residing in long-term care facilities is vulnerable not just because of reactivation from prior infection but also through acquisition of infection from other residents who develop disease [Thrupp et al. 2004].

Healthcare personnel in the United States have been shown to be at higher risk of acquiring TB than the general population [Menzies et al. 2007]. In the United States, multiple healthcare-associated TB outbreaks have been reported with patient-to-patient and patient-to-healthcare personnel transmission occurring [Cookson and Jarvis 1997]. TB disease outbreaks in long-term care facilities have also been reported [Stead 1981; Morris and Nell 1988; Ijaz et al. 2002; CDC 2012a]. Consistently, the most important factor favoring healthcare-associated transmission has been close contact with patients with unrecognized active TB disease [Craven et al. 1975; Catanzaro 1982; Kantor et al. 1988; Pearson et al. 1992; Griffith et al. 1995]. In our investigation, the TST and QFT-GIT conversions in the residents and employees of the secure access unit are likely attributed to the resident with active TB disease unrecognized until May 2012.

TB prevention and control in long-term care facilities has been difficult for several reasons. First, TB disease in older patients can present atypically and may not exhibit classic features. Many patients present clinically with changes in functional capacity, chronic fatigue, cognitive impairment, decreased appetite, or unexplained low-grade fever, symptoms which have a long differential diagnosis in the elderly [Nagami and Yoshikawa 1983; Yoshikawa 1992; Rajagopalan and Yoshikawa 2000]. Second, diagnosis in the elderly population in long-term care facilities is challenged by the occurrence of false negative TSTs, limited radiographic capabilities of these facilities, the difficulty in transporting residents to acute care centers for clinical evaluation, and the difficulty of obtaining expectorated sputum from cognitively impaired patients, as experienced by the facility in this evaluation [Thrupp et al. 2004]. Diagnosis may be hampered by end of life care decisions, and few long-term care facility deaths lead to autopsies [Katz and Seidel 1990]. Finally, many long-term care facilities do not have the capabilities for engineering and respiratory protection controls. Many facilities, including the one in our investigation, are not equipped with airborne infection isolation rooms for confirmed or suspected TB patients, nor do their employees participate in a respiratory protection program.

ANSI/ASHRAE has indicated that ventilation system design in skilled nursing homes is based on controlling odors, providing adequate filtration, and controlling airflow between certain areas. It is not as critical to control general bacteria levels (not *M. tuberculosis*) as compared to acute care hospitals [ASHRAE 2011]. However, ASHRAE recommends that central ventilation and air-conditioning systems in nursing facilities be fitted with at least one MERV 14 filter in resident care, treatment, diagnostic, and related areas to help reduce bacterial load in the air. This facility provided MERV 8 filtration of recirculated air. ASHRAE does not have a recommendation for the pressure relationship between resident rooms and adjacent areas, nor does it specifically recommend that air from resident rooms be exhausted directly outside [ASHRAE 2011]. This facility did exhaust air from resident rooms directly outside in some areas, while other areas recirculated return air, mixed with 40% outdoor air. ASHRAE does recommend maintaining bathrooms in nursing homes under negative pressure relative to adjacent areas [ASHRAE 2011]. We noted that for a few bathrooms, this was not always the case.

ANSI/ASHRAE recommends that the indoor CO_2 concentration be within 700 ppm of the outdoor concentration for comfort (odor) reasons [ANSI/ASHRAE 2010]. CO_2 is a normal constituent of exhaled breath and is not considered a building air pollutant. It is an indicator of whether sufficient quantities of outdoor air are being introduced into an occupied space. ASHRAE [2011] recommends that the temperature in nursing homes be maintained at 75°F throughout the building in the summer, and 75°F in resident rooms and 70°F in nonresident areas in winter. ASHRAE also recommends that RH should be maintained at 50% in summer, when air conditioning systems are used, but does not provide an RH recommendation for winter conditions, indicating that the RH levels "are best left to the judgment of the designers." At this facility, temperatures ranged from 74°F–83°F in the nursing station areas, and RH ranged from 18%–34%.

Though the comfort parameters collected in the minimum dataset office either met or were close to ANSI/ASHRAE guidelines, the reported "stuffiness" in the office is not unexpected given the small size of the office for the number of employees. Further evaluation of the ventilation in this office should be done. ANSI/ASHRAE [2010b] recommends outdoor air supply rates of 5 cubic feet per minute/person for office spaces.

Conclusions

A health hazard from exposure to *M. tuberculosis* existed at this long-term care facility. Extensive TB screening of residents and employees by the facility and supporting agencies through interviews, TST and QFT-GIT testing, chest radiographs, and sputum collection for AFB analysis revealed 12 residents and 16 employees with latent TB infection and one resident with active TB disease. No other sources of active TB disease were identified though several potential explanations for transmission existed. Because no further TST or QFT-GIT conversions have been identified since April 2012, it appears that TB transmission has stopped.

Recommendations

On the basis of our findings, we recommend the actions listed below to create a more healthful workplace. We encourage the long-term care facility to use a labor-management health and safety committee or working group to discuss the recommendations in this report and develop an action plan. Those involved in the work can best set priorities and assess the feasibility of our recommendations for the specific situation at the medical center. Our recommendations are based on the hierarchy of controls approach according to CDC guidelines [CDC 2005]. This approach groups actions by their likely effectiveness in reducing or removing hazards. We acknowledge that this facility is limited with the extent of its respiratory protection controls because it does not provide care for residents with airborne infectious disease. Therefore, we focus on administrative and engineering controls.

More comprehensive recommendations can be found in CDC's "Guidelines for Preventing the Transmission of *Mycobacterium tuberculosis* in Health-Care Settings, 2005" at http://www.cdc.gov/mmwr/preview/mmwrhtml/rr5417a1.htm?s_cid=rr5417a1_e [CDC 2005] and the Society for Healthcare Epidemiology of America's position paper titled "Tuberculosis Prevention and Control in Long-Term-Care Facilities for Older Adults" [Thrupp et al. 2004].

Administrative Controls

The most important level of TB controls is the use of administrative measures to reduce the risk for exposure to persons who might have TB disease [CDC 2005]. Administrative controls are management-dictated work practices and policies to reduce or prevent exposures to workplace hazards. The effectiveness of administrative changes in work practices for controlling workplace hazards is dependent on management commitment and employee acceptance. Regular monitoring and reinforcement are necessary to ensure that control policies and procedures are not circumvented in the name of convenience.

1. Provide general TB training during working hours to all employees on hire and annually thereafter to ensure a thorough understanding of the disease, its transmission, and ways to prevent it. Training for employees with direct resident contact should include the procedures for residents known or suspected of having active TB disease and for reporting healthcare personnel exposure to a resident with active TB disease. Training should be tailored to education level and clinical role. Training specific for long-term care facility staff titled "Preventing TB in Long-term Care" can be found on the OSHA website at http://www.osha.gov/dte/grant_materials/fy05/46c4-ht27/manual_english.pdf. Other general training and education materials can be found on the CDC TB website at http://www.cdc.gov/tb/.

2. Monitor current south side residents clinically for signs and symptoms of active TB disease at least once a month. Arrange prompt clinical evaluation for any resident with signs and symptoms of active TB disease, as feasible and clinically appropriate.

3. Instruct all employees to report signs and symptoms of active TB disease in residents to the caring physician and Medical Director immediately. As per the facility's tuberculosis plan, a resident with suspected disease should be transferred to an acute care facility within 5 hours of recognition.

4. Continue TST or QFT-GIT placement and symptom screening of all south side residents, employees, and direct care volunteers at least every 6 months. The screening interval may return to every year if conditions are met as outlined according to the TB risk assessment and recommendations in the CDC guidelines [CDC 2005]. Enforce the requirement for employee TB screening. Enforcement methods could include disabling privileges to electronic health records or disabling access to resident care areas. Arrange prompt clinical evaluation for any residents, employees, or volunteers with signs and symptoms of active TB disease or TST or QFT-GIT conversion. Offer treatment for latent TB infection to residents, employees, and volunteers once active TB disease has been ruled out.

5. Consider screening regular entertainer volunteers for TB through the employee health clinic prior to starting volunteer activities and annually thereafter.

6. Preserve visitors' log sheets for at least 6 months not only to detect unknown active TB disease cases but also to facilitate a contact investigation should a current resident be diagnosed with active TB disease. Require visitors to sign in upon entry to the facility.

Engineering Controls

Engineering controls are the second line of defense in the TB infection control program [CDC 2005]. Engineering controls prevent the spread and reduce the concentration of airborne *Mycobacterium tuberculosis* in ambient air. These technologies include local exhaust, ventilation, general ventilation, high-efficiency particulate air filtration, and ultraviolet germicidal irradiation. Engineering controls are very effective in protecting employees without placing primary responsibility of implementation on the employee. We realize that residents will be moved into the new facility this year. Therefore, some of our recommendations may only apply if the areas we evaluated are still in use.

1. Upgrade the ventilation system to provide MERV 14 filtration for resident areas according to ASHRAE guidelines [2011]. Most ventilation systems are designed to handle specific filters. Consult a ventilation engineer familiar with nursing home ventilation design before making filtration changes in your ventilation system.

2. Increase exhaust ventilation in bathrooms that were observed to have bidirectional airflow. Test and balance all other bathroom exhaust ventilation in the building to ensure that airflow is directed into bathrooms according to ASHRAE guidelines [2011].

3. Maintain temperature according to ASHRAE guidelines for nursing homes [ASHRAE 2011].

4. Consult a ventilation engineer to further evaluate the minimum dataset office. In the interim, add a relief vent to the minimum dataset office doorway to the adjacent hallway to facilitate additional air exchange between these two areas and alleviate stuffiness complaints from employees in this area.

References

ANSI/ASHRAE [2010a]. Thermal environmental conditions for human occupancy. American National Standards Institute/ASHRAE standard 55-2010. Atlanta, GA: American Society for Heating, Refrigerating, and Air-Conditioning Engineers.

ANSI/ASHRAE [2010b]. Ventilation for acceptable indoor air quality. American National Standards Institute/ASHRAE standard 62.1-2010. Atlanta, GA: American Society of Heating, Refrigerating, and Air-Conditioning Engineers, Inc.

ASHRAE [2011]. Health-care facilities. In: 2011 ASHRAE Handbook - HVAC Applications. I-P Edition. Atlanta, GA: American Society for Heating, Refrigerating, and Air-Conditioning Engineers, Inc., pp. 8.14–8.15.

Catanzaro A [1982]. Nosocomial tuberculosis. Am Rev Respir Dis *125*(5):559–562.

Cookson ST, Jarvis WR [1997]. Prevention of nosocomial transmission of *Mycobacterium tuberculosis*. Infect Dis Clin North Am *11*(2):385–409.

CDC (Centers for Disease Control and Prevention) [1990]. Prevention and control of tuberculosis in facilities providing long-term care to the elderly (ACET). MMWR *39* (RR–10).

CDC [2005]. Guidelines for preventing transmission of *Mycobacterium tuberculosis* in health-care settings. MMWR *54*(RR-17):1–141.

CDC [2012a]. Notes from the field: tuberculosis outbreak in a long-term-care facility for mentally ill persons — Puerto Rico, 2010–2012. MMWR *61*(39):801.

CDC [2012b]. Reported tuberculosis in the United States, 2011. Atlanta, GA: U.S. Department of Health and Human Services, CDC, October 2012. [http://www.cdc.gov/tb/statistics/reports/2011/pdf/report2011.pdf]. Date accessed: May 2013.

Craven RB, Wenzel RL, Atuk NO [1975]. Minimizing tuberculosis risk to hospital personnel and students exposed to unsuspected disease. Ann Intern Med *82*(5):628–632.

Griffith DE, Hardeman JL, Zhang Y, Wallace RJ, Mazurek GH [1995]. Tuberculosis outbreak among healthcare workers in a community hospital. Am J Respir Crit Care Med *152*(2):808–811.

Ijaz K, Dillaha JA, Yang Z, Cave MD, Bates JH [2002]. Unrecognized tuberculosis in a nursing home causing death with spread of tuberculosis to the community. J Am Geriatr Soc *50*(7):1213–1218.

Kantor HS, Poblete R, Pusateri SL [1988]. Nosocomial transmission of tuberculosis from unsuspected disease. Am J Med *84*(5):833–838.

Katz PR, Seidel G [1990]. Nursing home autopsies. Survey of physician attitudes and practice patterns. Arch Pathol Lab Med *114*(2):145–147.

Menzies D, Joshi R, Pai M [2007]. Risk of tuberculosis infection and disease associated with work in health care settings. Int J Tuberc Lung Dis *11*(6):593–605.

Morris CD, Nell H [1988]. Epidemic of pulmonary tuberculosis in geriatric homes. S Afr Med J *74*(3):117–120.

Nagami P, Yoshikawa TT [1983]. Tuberculosis in the geriatric patient. J Am Geriatr Soc *31*(6):356–363.

Pearson ML, Jereb JA, Frieden TR, Crawford JT, Davis BJ, Dooley SW, Jarvis WR [1992]. Nosocomial transmission of multidrug-resistant *Mycobacterium tuberculosis*. Ann Intern Med *117*(3):191–196.

Rajagopalan S, Yoshikawa TT [2000]. Tuberculosis in long-term-care facilities. Infect Control Hosp Epidemiol *21*(9):611–615.

Stead WW [1981]. Tuberculosis among elderly persons: an outbreak in a nursing home. Ann Intern Med *94*(5):606–610.

Thrupp L, Bradley S, Smith P, Simor A, Gantz N, Crossley K, Loeb M, Strausbaugh L, Nicolle L, SHEA Long-Term-Care Committee [2004]. Tuberculosis prevention and control in long-term-care facilities for older adults. Infect Control Hosp Epidemiol *25*(12):1097–1108.

Yoshikawa TT [1992]. Tuberculosis in aging adults. J Am Geriatr Soc *40*(2):178–187.

Keywords: NAICS 623110 (Nursing Care Facilities [Skilled Nursing Facilities]), tuberculosis, *Mycobacterium tuberculosis*, long-term care, nursing home

The Health Hazard Evaluation Program investigates possible health hazards in the workplace under the authority of Section 20(a)(6) of the Occupational Safety and Health Act of 1970, 29 U.S.C. 669(a)(6). The Health Hazard Evaluation Program also provides, upon request, technical assistance to federal, state, and local agencies to control occupational health hazards and to prevent occupational illness and disease. Regulations guiding the Program can be found in Title 42, Code of Federal Regulations, Part 85; Requests for Health Hazard Evaluations (42 CFR 85).

Acknowledgments

Desktop Publishers: Mary Winfree
Editor: Ellen Galloway
Health Communicator: Stefanie Brown
Logistics: Donnie Booher and Karl Feldmann
Medical Field Assistance: Judith Eisenberg; David Jackson, University of Cincinnati College of Medicine; and Kimberly Porter and Donna Fearey, Alaska Department of Health and Social Services
Subject Matter Consultation: Robert Luo, Sundari Mase, and Kiren Mitruka, NCHHSTP

Availability of Report

This report is available at http://www.cdc.gov/niosh/hhe/reports/pdfs/2012-0137-3178.pdf.

Recommended citation for this report:
NIOSH [2013]. Health hazard evaluation report: evaluation of exposure to tuberculosis among employees at a long-term care facility. By de Perio MA, Niemeier RT. Cincinnati, OH: U.S. Department of Health and Human Services, Centers for Disease Control and Prevention, National Institute for Occupational Safety and Health, NIOSH HETA No. 2012-0137-3178.